Heart Failure and *You*

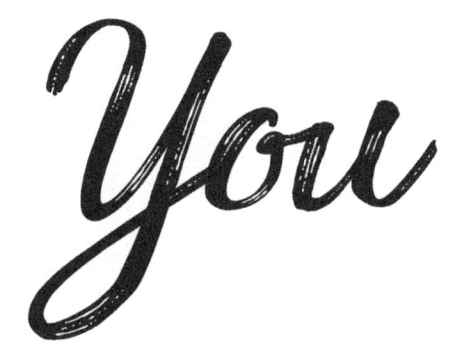

A Practical Guide for Managing Your Heart Health

CASS THOMPSON

© 2023 Cassandra Thompson

All rights reserved. No part of this book may be reproduced in any form or by electronic or mechanical means, including information storage and retrieval systems, without written permission from the author, except for the use of brief quotations in critical articles or reviews.

ISBN (paperback): 9798868482038

Disclaimer.

The information and suggestions in this book are based on the author's research and personal professional experience. They are not intended as a substitute for consulting with a physician or healthcare provider. The publisher and authors are not responsible for any adverse effects or consequences from using any suggestions, preparations, or exercises discussed in this book. The information is general and intended to better inform readers of their diet and healthcare choices. You should always consult your physician or healthcare provider regarding any changes you plan to make to your health, diet, or exercise regimen.

Written and Published by

Cassandra Thompson

Editing by

Tammy Kling

BookBaby

Contributing Author

Patricia A. Joines RN, BSN

Content Reviewers

Stephanie C. Hodges MS-ENS

Carmen Nolan RN, NP

Book Cover Design

Elena L1 Graphics

Layout design

Chaker Lahmadi @iligantdesign

*Dedicated to my dad,
Elton Thompson Sr.*

Dear reader,

I hope you find the information on the following pages a valuable resource guide for your heart failure journey. I wrote this book as a healthcare professional and the daughter of someone with heart failure. I lost my father due to poorly managed health conditions resulting from not managing his heart failure effectively. It's hard to lose someone to something that could have been prevented, so I feel strongly about helping others get a head start in preventing common complications of heart failure.

I want to educate and help as many people as possible by providing a basic understanding of heart failure with a small set of tools that can be used to manage their current heart failure condition, prevent other heart-related issues, and avoid any progression of the disease. Please know that you are not alone wherever you are on your journey. **We are all in this together.**

BOOK CONTENTS

CHAPTER 1

- Your Heart Health
- Heart Healthy Eating
- Meal Prepping

CHAPTER 2

- Monitoring your sodium intake
- Monitoring your fluid restriction
- Sodium Conversion Table
- Fluid Conversion Table

CHAPTER 3

- Working Out for Your Heart
- Blood Pressure and Weight
- Red Flags

- Conclusion
- Personal Information
- Medical Information
- Medications
- References

INTRODUCTION

Being diagnosed with heart failure can be challenging to navigate and understand. If you've ever had any experience with a family member with heart failure or faced it yourself, you are aware of the complex issues surrounding it.

Heart failure is something that I am familiar with, both personally and professionally. I've encountered people with different ideas about managing heart failure based on their understanding of what the diagnosis means to them. Some approach this with a complete understanding of what it will take to manage their heart failure successfully. At the same time, others struggle with one misconception after the other.

As an emergency room nurse, I see patients during the early onset of heart failure and when they have not managed their condition effectively. Often, it is because people focus solely on following their medication regimen and not their diet, fluid, and sodium restrictions.

But what if there were no prescription medications available to treat heart failure? Then, patients would focus on diet and exercise. Society has been conditioned to rely on medication as the sole solution for years. Medication is necessary for managing the disease, but diet and exercise are also essential to managing heart failure successfully.

Most people with heart failure don't fully understand the fluid and sodium restrictions. Both will require you to cut back on processed foods and limit the intake of fruits and vegetables, which seems contradictory because it's easy to think that eating a salad or bowl of fruit is better than eating a hot dog or a turkey sandwich.

Now, this isn't to say that you can't or shouldn't eat a bowl of fruit, a salad, or a turkey sandwich; this is just to raise awareness about how they will affect your fluid and sodium intake.

With the number of people in the United States living with heart failure being more than six million, according to the CDC (Centers for Disease Control and Prevention), I think it's high time we try to learn more about the disease, understand how to manage it more effectively and take control of our heart health. **If we can tackle this, we can extend life.**

"Don't compromise yourself, you're all you've got."

JANIS JOPLIN

CHAPTER 1
HEART FACTS

1. A healthy heart pumps 2,000 gallons of blood through your body daily.

2. The heart weighs less than one pound.

3. The heart beats about 100,000 times a day.

4. There are 60,000 miles of blood vessels in the body.

5. Intense and sudden feelings of sadness can mimic the symptoms of a heart attack.

"Conversely, laughter is good for the heart!
Think of ways to add more laughter to your life."

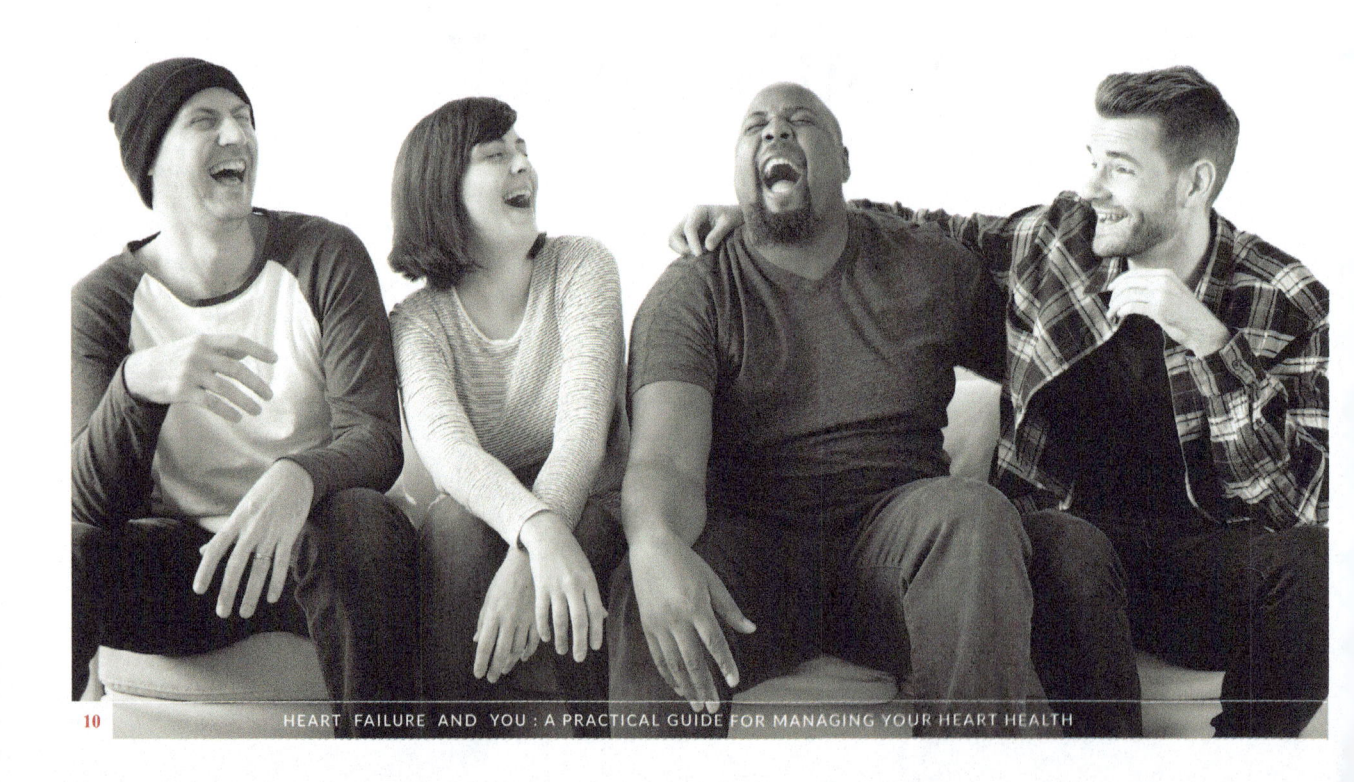

YOUR HEART HEALTH

A good hearty laugh increases the heart rate and the number of breaths taken. This seamless action enhances the body's oxygen flow, circulation, and vascular function. As a result, your mood is improved, anxiety is relieved, and elevated blood pressure is decreased.

An article written by Dr. Karthikeyan Anath of Henry Ford Health Cardiology discusses how emotions can negatively and positively affect your heart and how laughing can help the body fight off illnesses. He explains how stress hormones caused by anger can cause inflammation and muscle spasms that can trigger a heart attack. Additionally, hormones released by anxiety or stress can increase the risk of decreased blood flow and circulation, leading to heart disease.

We have all heard of elderly people who "died of heartbreak" after their spouse passed, and if that is true, the opposite should be as well. Happiness, laughter, and joyful people should contribute to our healing! For example, laughter reduces the body's cortisol levels, burns calories, and, best of all, those feel-good hormones called endorphins are released. (Karthikeyan Ananth, 2019)

Isn't it exciting to learn that laughter can improve heart health and reduce the risk of heart disease?

"Laughter is good for the soul?"

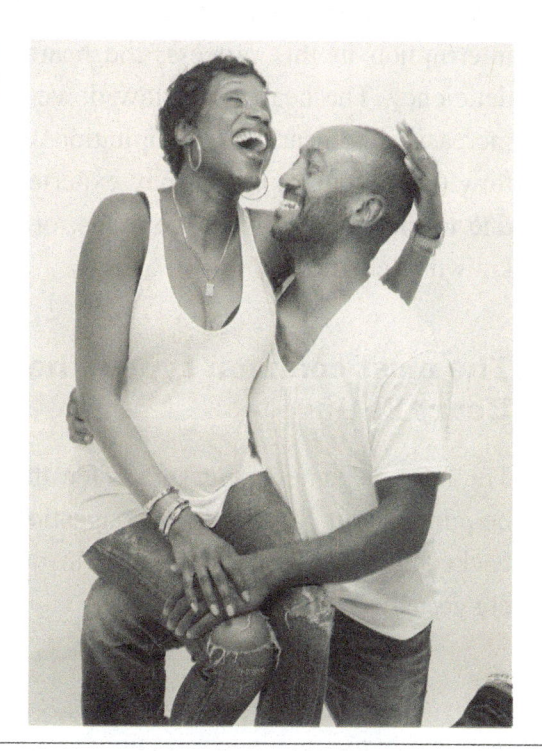

HEART FAILURE BASICS

Heart failure occurs when the heart can no longer pump blood and oxygen throughout the body or fill up with blood efficiently due to slow heart muscle contractions.

The most common cause of heart failure is:

- High blood pressure and high cholesterol that are not managed effectively.
- Heart valves that do not open and close properly.
- Heart muscle infection.
- Lung disease.
- Heart attack.
- Some chemotherapy medications.

Heart failure is typically a long-term (chronic) condition that affects multiple organs in the body. The heart should work effortlessly, much like breathing. If there is an interruption in this process, the heart will try to compensate or make up for the deficiency. The heart may slow down the time it takes to refill after it contracts by increasing the heartbeats (palpitations). It may increase size (enlarge) to allow blood flow (cardiomegaly). You may experience shortness of breath or difficulty breathing due to increased fluid in the lungs, or you may experience lower leg swelling, also known as edema.

The most common type of heart failure is called Congestive Heart Failure.

The heart becomes congested when the blood returns to the heart faster than it can be pumped out. Think of the congestion like a traffic jam. Once the main roadway is backed up, it causes delays on the surrounding roads, which leads to the area becoming congested.

Normal Heart   **Congestive Heart**

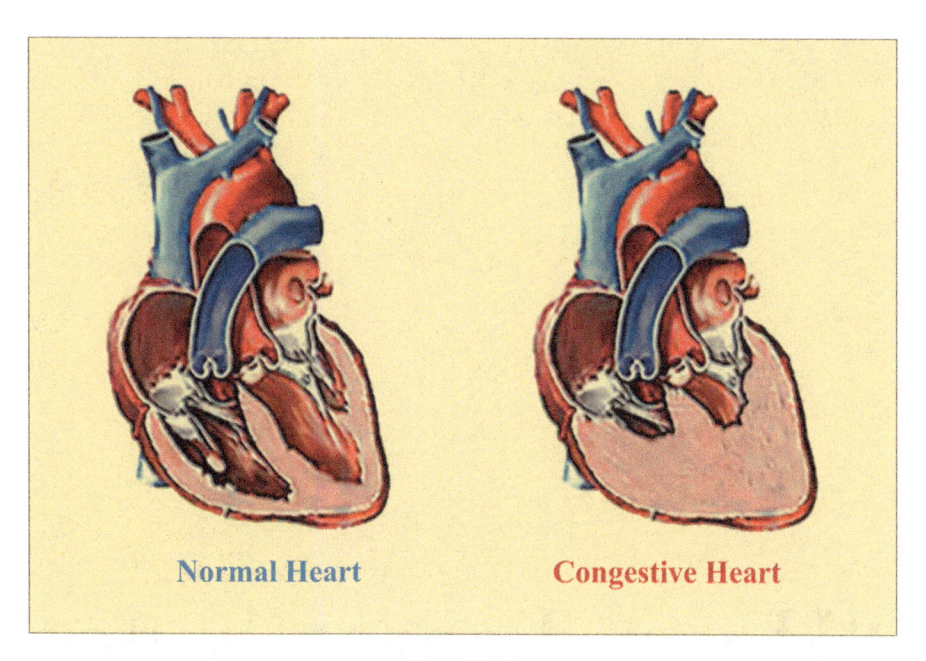

(Jayan 2019)

When you have congestive heart failure (CHF), there is also reduced blood supply to the kidneys, resulting in water and sodium retention. The kidneys filter over fifty gallons of blood every twenty-four hours, with the heart providing roughly 25%. CHF reduces the kidneys' ability to filter blood, aid in controlling blood pressure, and remove waste through urine. If your heart failure is not managed effectively, this will eventually lead to renal failure.

But all is not lost; the disease progression of heart failure can significantly be decreased and, in some cases, be reversed with the right treatment plan.

"Heart disease is not
a death sentence;
it's a wake-up call."

WILLIAM MARKS

HEART HEALTHY EATING

Whether you are diagnosed with heart failure in a clinical setting or emergency room, you will be referred to a cardiologist. During that visit, you will be given a treatment plan based on your type of heart failure and the severity of the disease. Treatment plans generally consist of a cardiac-specific diet, fluid and sodium restriction, instructions on blood pressure and weight management, and an exercise plan.

The cardiologist will briefly explain the diet changes you'll need to make and the restrictions on your daily fluid and sodium intake. The nurse or dietician will then review the diet changes and restrictions with you, asking, throughout the visit, if you have any questions.

Unfortunately, most patients and family members aren't sure what questions to ask after being given a ton of information to process. They leave the doctor's office without understanding what they should or should not eat or what a daily fluid and sodium intake restriction is.

Most people get the gist of the cardiac diet. They understand that the goal is to eat lots of fruits and vegetables, whole grains, lean poultry, and fish high in omega-3 fatty acids. And to avoid eating fried fatty foods and to limit their sugar intake.

They understand that the sodium restriction means avoiding salt; however, that is only part of decreasing the sodium intake. Sodium is practically in everything that we eat and drink.

Most people only associate fluid with what they drink. Again, that is only part of our fluid intake. It also includes fruits, vegetables, and quite a few pantry items.

People always say, "I would eat healthier if I could afford it," or "I would cook more if I had time." The key to eating healthy is knowing how to do it cost-effectively without spending an entire day in the kitchen prepping and cooking. With the right plan and preparation, eating healthy is less expensive and requires less time in the kitchen.

Eating a heart-healthy diet isn't just good for your heart; it improves cholesterol, balances blood pressure, controls blood sugar, and helps you maintain a healthy body weight.

The goal is to make small changes in your thought process of approaching food and changing your perspective on shopping for and preparing food.

Most people say that you eat first with your eyes; it's not just about the food being visually appealing, but people tend to put more food on their plate when they see they have more food options. And they tend to buy more food at the grocery store when they shop hungry.

You'll also often hear people say, "My eyes are bigger than my stomach." Well, an empty stomach is about the size of your fist, and the brain has a funny way of making you think your stomach is bigger than it is. When you eat, the stomach expands, and it can hold about a quart of food without making you feel like you overate; two to four quarts and we start to feel like we ate more than we should have.

Learning to eat healthy is just as much about knowing what to eat as it is about how much to eat. According to the American Diabetes Association's article on Healthy Eating, by using the "Diabetes Plate Method," "you can create perfectly portioned meals with a healthy balance of vegetables, protein, and carbohydrates." (Recipes and Nutrition 2020)

Use a small plate or bowl instead of a standard-size plate to control your portion size. Your serving size should consist of 50% vegetables, 25% carbohydrates, 25% protein, and a glass of water or a low-calorie drink.

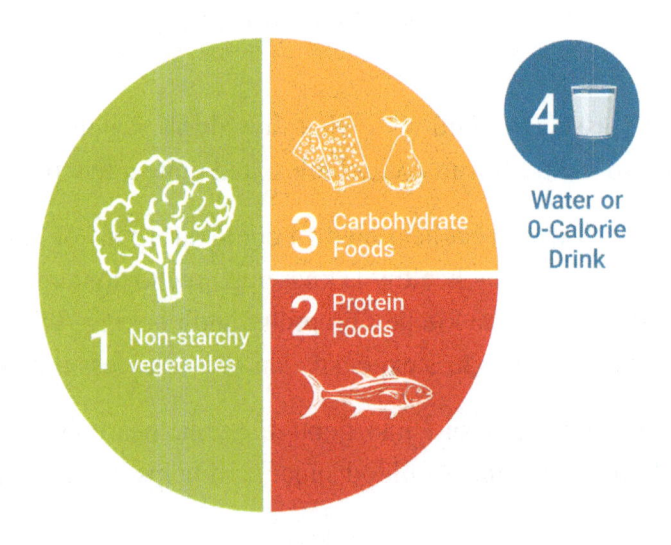

Prepping your meals beforehand will also allow you to control what and how much you eat. Your meal prep container should be 50% vegetables and 50% protein. Plan out weekly menus and pick two days out of the week to prep and cook your meals. Remember to include snacks.

Learning how to break years of diet and eating habits in a short period of time is going to be overwhelming at first but making small changes a little at a time will make it easier to start and maintain. Your life depends on it. You have to learn how to balance what you can eat and drink with what and how much you have to limit.

And hey, we're all human, so don't beat yourself up if you eat something that is not considered "heart healthy;" it's okay to allow yourself a treat occasionally. It won't ruin your heart-healthy diet. Just spread your treat days out, and don't gift yourself with one regularly.

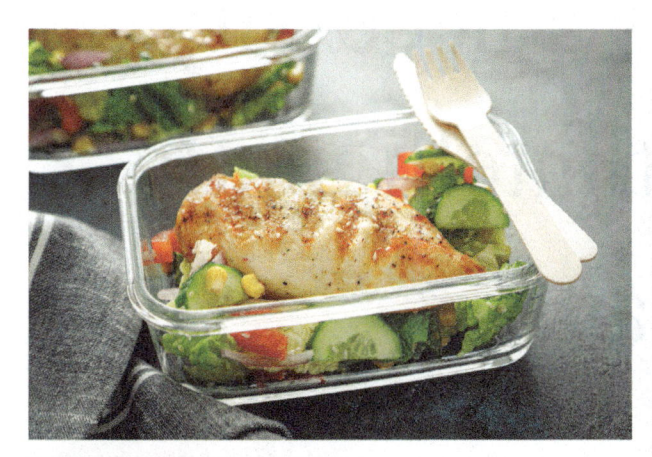

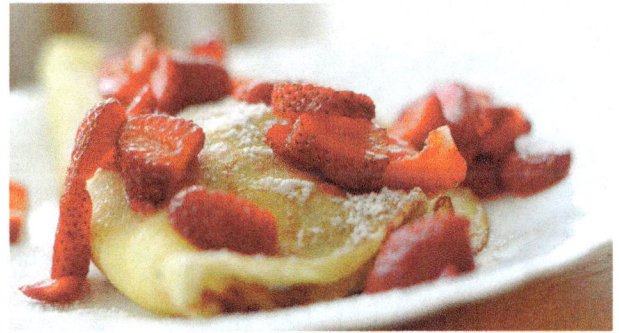

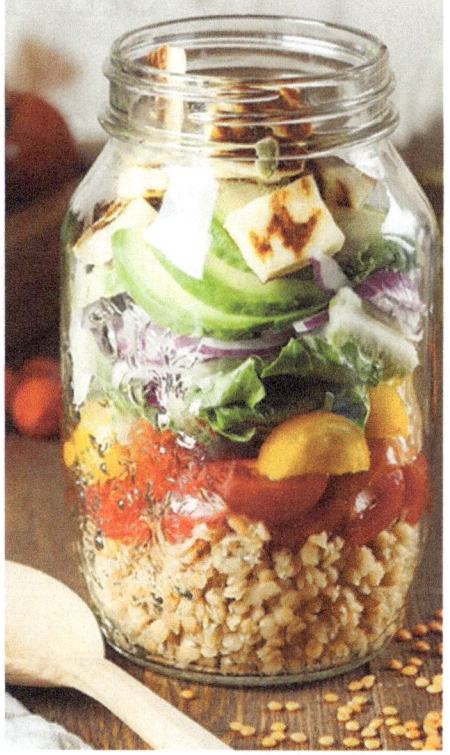

> "To eat is a necessity,
> but to eat intelligently
> is an art"

— LA ROCHEFOUCAULD

MEAL PREP TIPS

Meal prepping for breakfast, lunch, dinner, and snacks once or twice a week will save you time and money. Whether you buy groceries once a month or once weekly, the key is only to buy what you plan to eat for one to two weeks. Invest in freezer bags, meal prep containers, and mason jars.

When putting together your meal plan, include lots of vegetables, lean protein meats, or plant-based proteins. Carbs aren't necessary, but if you want to add them to your meal plan, carbs and grains should only account for 25% of your meal prep container.

Also, frozen vegetables are as good as fresh vegetables, and you get more bang for your buck. For instance, you can get a 16oz bag of frozen vegetables for less than $2.50 and split that one bag into four meal prep dishes.

Choose cooking oils such as canola or avocado for pan frying and sautéing. Use extra-virgin olive oil for sauces and vinaigrettes. Canola, avocado, and EVO oils are heart-healthy monounsaturated fats.

· **Green vegetables and root vegetables are rich in folate and potassium.**
Examples include kale, spinach, collards, cabbage, carrots, sweet potatoes, and turnips.

· **Lean proteins are low in saturated fat.**
Examples include fish, shellfish, turkey, skinless chicken, pork tenderloin

· **Plant-based proteins are low in fat and full of calcium and fiber.**
Examples include tofu, edamame, beans, lentils, quinoa.

Make the switch to wheat bread, brown sugar, and brown rice. They are higher in fiber, rich in vitamins such as folic acid, B6, and E, and minerals including chromium, magnesium, and zinc.

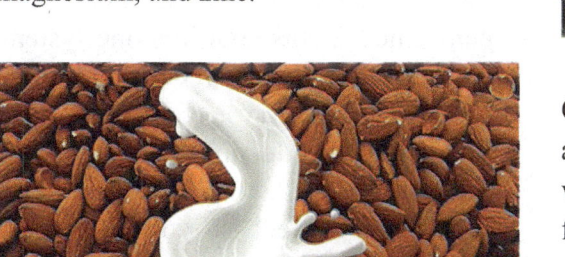

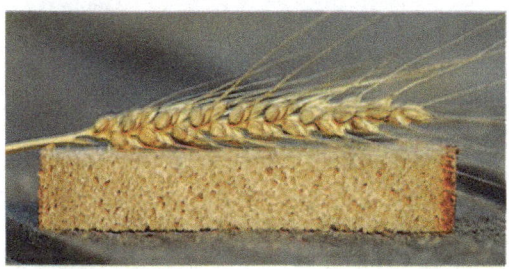

Choose a nut milk, such as almond or an oat milk. You're getting the protein, vitamins, and minerals without saturated fats and less sugar and carbs than whole milk.

For breakfast, try oatmeal breakfast cups. Start by cooking your oatmeal, scoop it into a muffin pan, top it off with your favorite topping, and toss it in the freezer. Once frozen, take them out of the pan, put the individual cups into a zip-lock bag, and put them back in the freezer. Now you've got breakfast for the week.

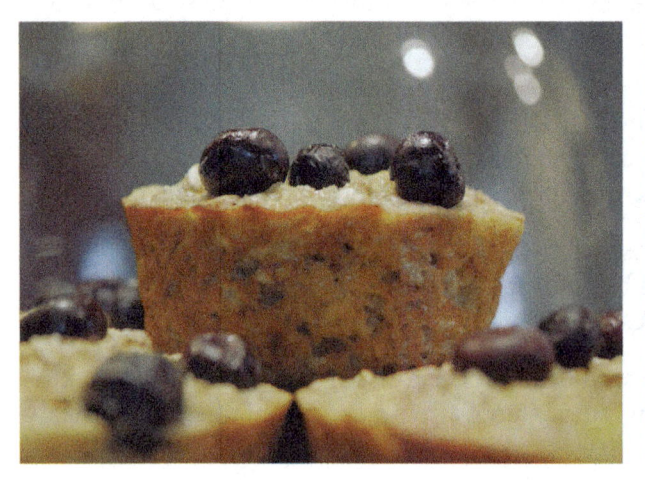

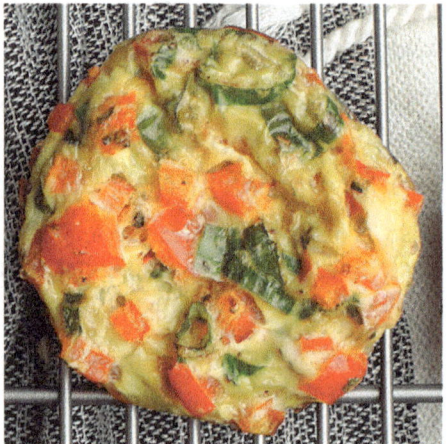

You can also use the same steps using grits or eggs. I like to make egg cups with peppers, onions, and spinach. Prepare your eggs just as you would if you were going to pan-fry them, but instead, fill your muffin pan tins and bake at 350 for about twenty minutes or so. Please make sure that all your cooked foods have completely cooled before freezing.

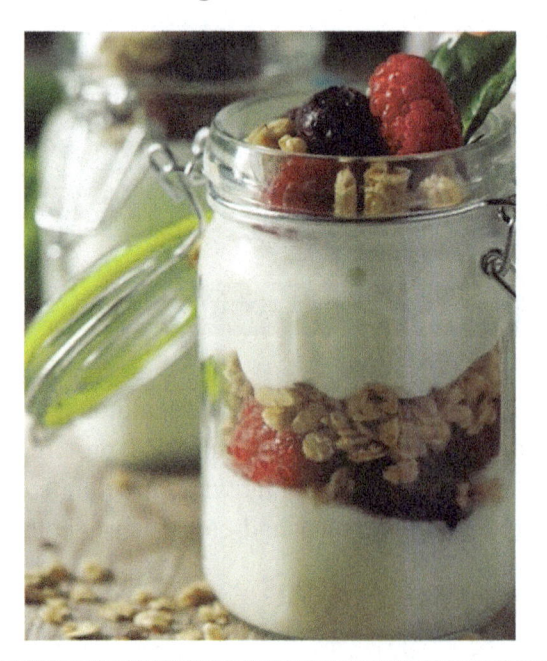

Yogurt fruit parfaits are great for breakfast, lunch, or a snack on the go. It's no secret that yogurt is good for our gut health, but did you know that Greek yogurt is high in protein, low in carbs, and contains vitamin B12 and zinc?

Protein is beneficial for tissue and muscle repair. Zinc benefits your immune system. B12 benefits red blood cell formation, improves nervous system function and boosts energy production. (Jillian Kubala 2021) Just be aware that yogurt can have a high sugar content, so you want to be mindful of the amount of sugar per serving when choosing your yogurt options.

For dinner, you can prepare your protein, vegetables, and starch options individually or make one-pot meals lasting up to three or four days.

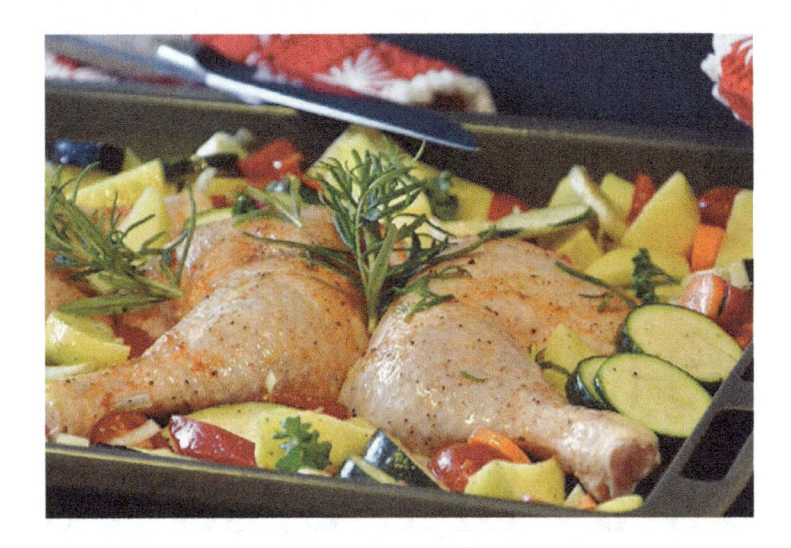

Invest in an air fryer. Your heart will thank you for it. It's so much healthier than frying your food in cooking oil. When you choose the option to air fry, you're cutting the calories by more than 50% and significantly decreasing the amount of fat.

You can boil eggs, bake potatoes, turkey burgers, and sweet potato fries. Make crispy tortilla chips and croutons for salads. Bake chicken parmesan or fry your favorite fish.

Please note that using an air fryer is not meant to replace baking in the oven, cooking on the stove, or using your roaster for one-pot meals. It is merely a healthier cooking option for some of your favorite foods.

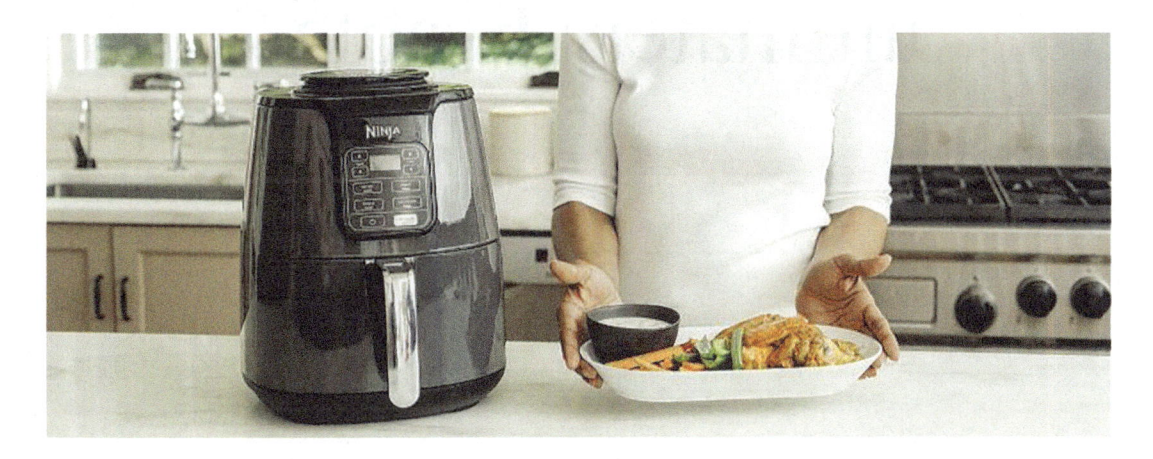

"Healthy eating is a way of life, so it's important to establish routines that are simple, realistically, and ultimately livable."

HORACE

CHAPTER 2

MONITORING YOUR SODIUM INTAKE

Sodium vs. salt, what's the difference? Sodium is found naturally in food or manufactured into processed foods, and salt is something we add to our food.

Sodium is a nutrient found in nearly everything you eat and drink, and it's essential to the human body. There is a daily recommended value of sodium, which is about 2,300 mg per day, and of that, around 500 mg of sodium is required to perform the necessary functions of transmitting nerve impulses, contracting, and relaxing muscles, and maintaining the body's water and mineral balance.

Most people diagnosed with heart failure are placed on a sodium restriction. The average restriction is typically 800 mg per day. Processed foods such as lunch meats, canned food products, frozen prepared meals, sugary desserts, sodas, and packaged foods have a very high sodium content. So, you'll want to limit your consumption or avoid them altogether.

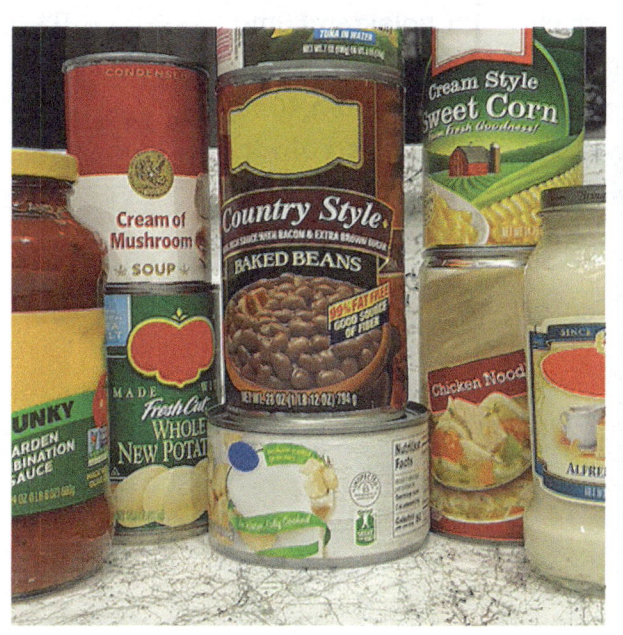

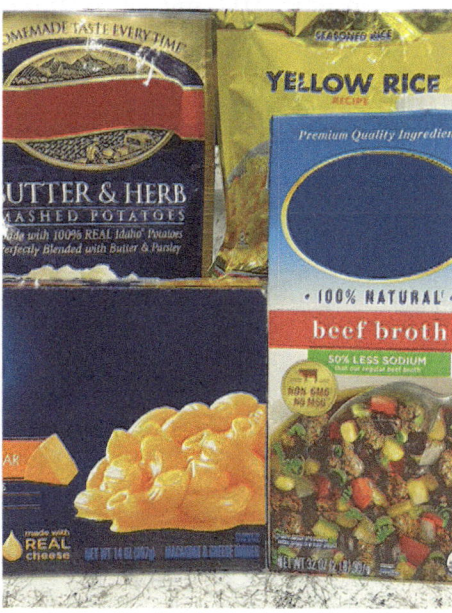

The most important step in watching your sodium intake will be to check the nutrition label.

There are four things that you are looking for on the nutrition label.

- Serving size per container
- Serving size
- Sodium
- Total Sugars

Let's assume that the recommended serving size is 1/2 cup, and it contains 400 mg of sodium and 17 gm of sugar. For every 1/2 cup you consume, you take in 400 mg of sodium. Therefore, if you have 1 cup, you will consume 800 mg of sodium, which might be your whole day's recommended sodium intake. You still have one or two other meals and snacks to consider, without any leeway. This is where innovative meal choices come in handy.

Nutrition Facts

Serving Size (33g)
Servings Per Container / Aprox 15

Amount Per Serving
Calories 160   Calories from Fat 70

	%Daily Value*
Total Fat 8g	12%
Saturated Fat 2.5g	13%
Trans Fat 0g	
Polyunsaturated Fat 2.5g	
Monounsaturated Fat 2g	
Cholesterol 0mg	0%
Sodium 110mg	5%
Potassium 40mg	1%
Total Carbohydrate	7%
Dietary Fiber less than	3%
Sugars 11g	

During a shopping trip with my dad, he wanted to get some lunch meat for a ham and turkey sandwich. So, we went to the lunch meat section to look at his options. I showed him how to calculate the sodium content in the ham and turkey per serving by checking the nutrition label.

A 9 oz package contains around 4.5 servings of thinly sliced deli lunchmeat. A package of ham has 2,565 mg of sodium and turkey has about 2,205 mg. The standard serving size for lunch meat is 2 oz, which equates to roughly four to six slices of thinly sliced deli lunch meat. For one serving of ham there is about 570 mg of sodium and turkey breast about 490 mg. However, calculating the sodium content didn't stop there. We also had to account for the sodium content in the bread, condiments, and cheese.

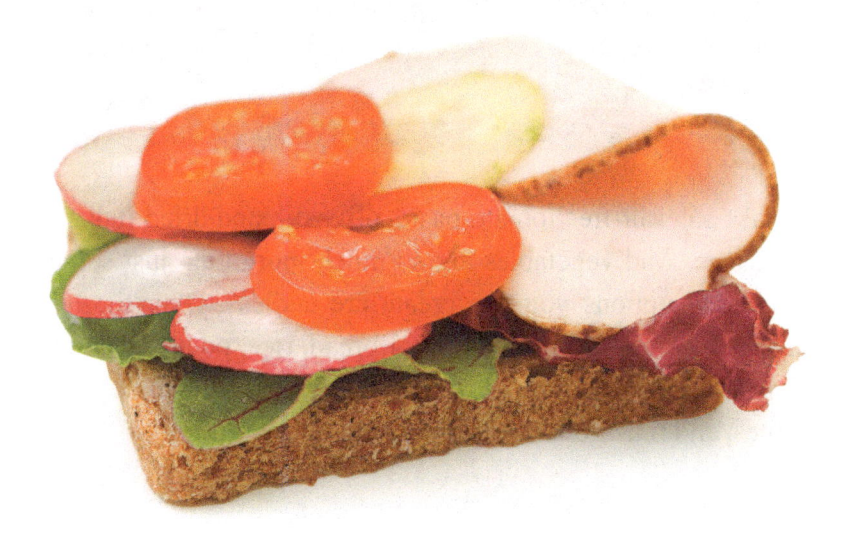

We calculated my dad's sandwich out to approximately 865mg of sodium with the turkey, but his restriction was limited to 800 mg. However, since he really wanted to eat the sandwich and I did not want to disappoint him, we compromised by making some adjustments. We removed the mayonnaise, cheese, one piece of meat, and a slice of bread which brought the sodium content down to around 500 mg. This allowed him to have an additional 300 mg of sodium for a snack and dinner which was within the permissible limit. And he was happy with that.

Pizza was another one of my dad's favorites, and pizza has anywhere from 1100 mg to 2300 mg of sodium per slice, making it very challenging to enjoy when you're on a sodium restriction. The good news is, Challenges create new experiences!

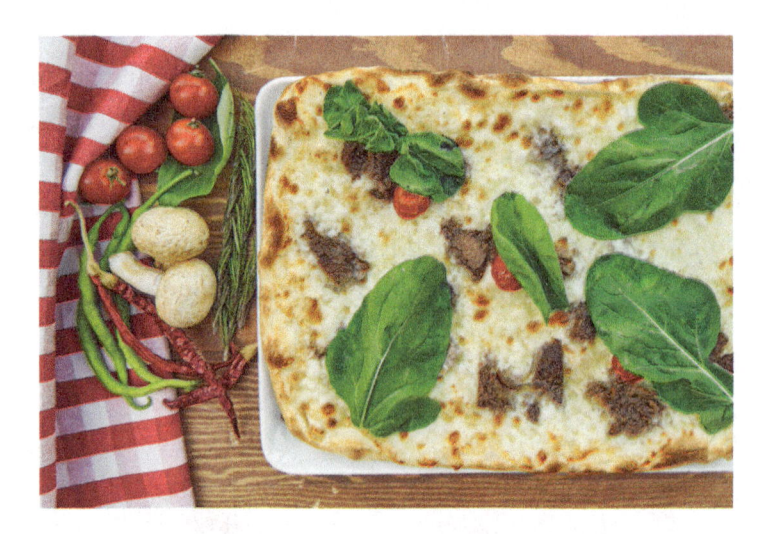

Let's make pizza! Grab salt-free tomato paste, olive oil, and dried Italian seasoning to make the pizza sauce. And vegetables are so much more than just something grown in a garden; the meal options you can create are endless. Over the last few years, cauliflower has been the go-to replacement for bread, rice, potatoes, and pasta. So, it's the perfect starter for making your pizza crust. Top it off with some skim mozzarella cheese, vegetables, and mushrooms as a meat substitute.

I am always on the lookout for new meal options for myself and my family. Since our dietary restrictions require low-sodium meals, I used to spend hours scouring the internet for recipes that fit our needs. With so many options available on Google, it was frustrating to find meals that met our requirements. Then I discovered Low SO Recipes, which has become my absolute favorite website. It offers a variety of visually appealing, delicious meal options that are easy to make with easy to find ingredients. The website is user-friendly, and the instructions are easy to follow. Kelly has recipes for everything from soups, salads, bread, pasta, sauces, and even ricotta cheese, and all of them are low sodium based.

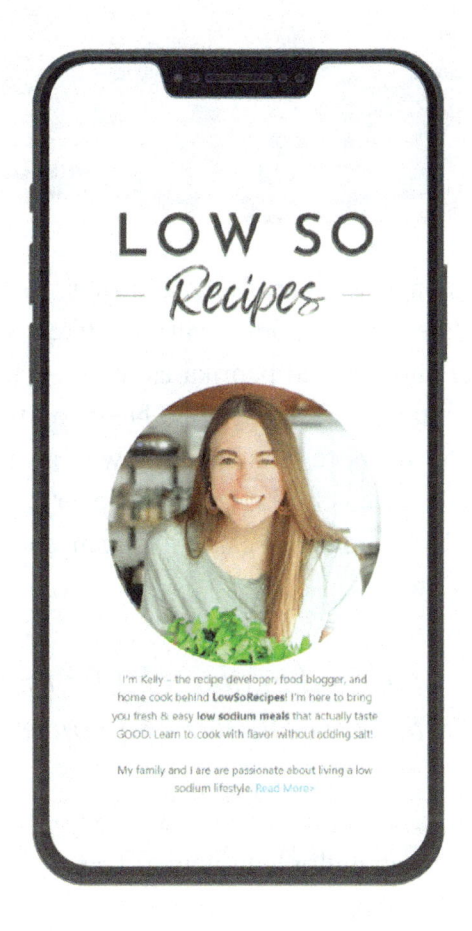

Website link: **https://lowsorecipes.com**

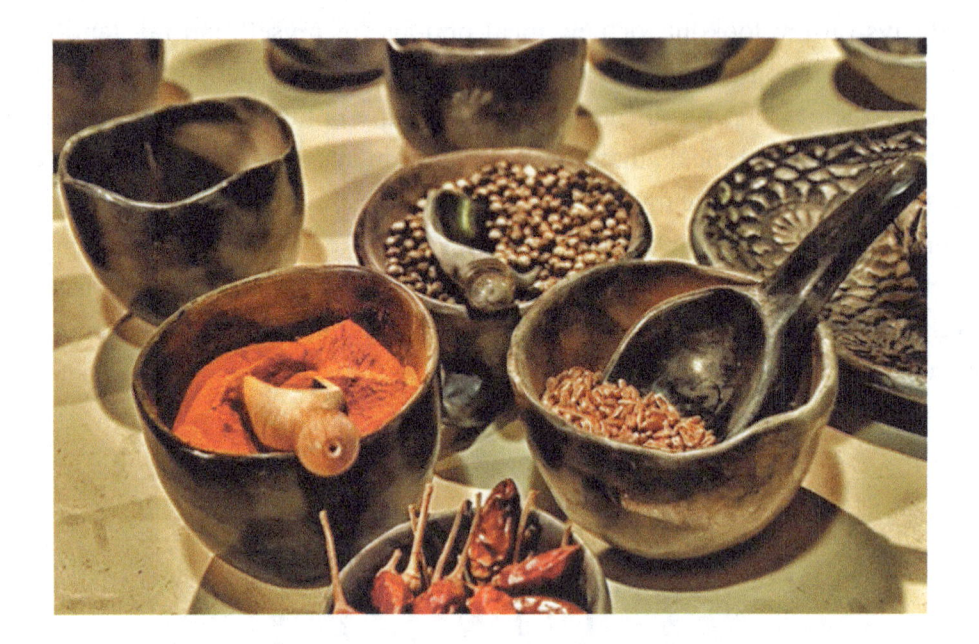

I also like to make my own seasoning blends and rubs. I start with a base seasoning based on my choice of protein or vegetables pairing. I like my meats on the spicier side, so I add cayenne pepper and smoked paprika as the base to those seasoning blends. With vegetables, I prefer Italian seasoning; I go heavy on the basil and parsley in the seasoning base. When I have a taste for something with a smokey flavor, I add cumin. But my personal favorite is dried chives; I add it to everything. Additionally, you can add aromatic vegetables like onions and garlic to enhance your dish's flavor or a spritz of citrus to enhance the taste.

> *The tongue is covered in about 8,000 taste buds, each containing up to 100 cells helping you taste your food.*

I've included a sample of a seasoning blend from one of the book's contributors that can be used in various ways on multiple protein or vegetables dishes, or you can use it as a template to create your own.

SMOKED RANCH SEASONING

Most of us have these items in our kitchen. You can use an empty mason jar, a large spice jar, or whatever airtight canister you have. My preference is a translucent glass jar, as seen in the photo.

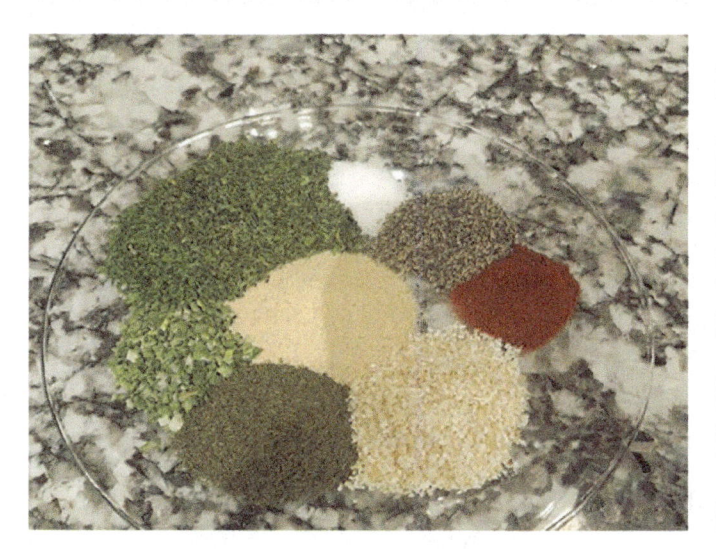

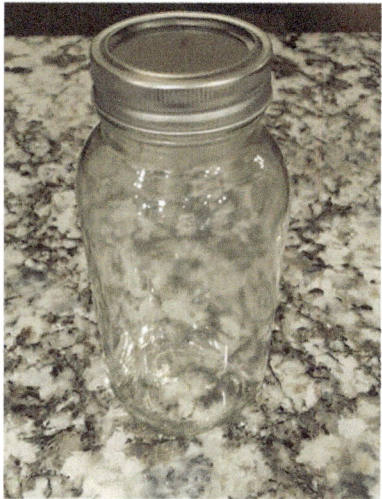

Gather all the ingredients listed below and put them in the jar as you go. I like to double the ingredients so I do not have to make more daily seasonings. You can use this seasoning as a marinade, adding extra virgin olive oil and vinegar to marinate your meat. I also use this seasoning to make homemade Italian and ranch dressing. You can sprinkle this seasoning on whatever you choose. It is so delicious. Have fun creating your favorite recipes with it! Use whichever brand you prefer or use fresh seasonings and dry them yourself using a dehydrator.

TWO VERSIONS

Low Sodium	Sodium-Free
You will need: • 4 Tablespoons of parsley. • ½ teaspoon of kosher fine or coarse sea salt or Himalayan pink salt. • 2 teaspoons of dried chives. • 4 teaspoons of garlic powder. • 4 teaspoons of onion powder. • 4 teaspoons of dried onion flakes. • 2 teaspoons of coarse ground black pepper. • 3 teaspoons of dill weed. • 1 Tablespoon of smoked paprika	You will need: • 4 Tablespoons of parsley. • 2 teaspoons of dried or freeze-dried chives. • 4 teaspoons of garlic powder. • 4 teaspoons of onion powder. • 4 teaspoons of dried onion flakes. • 2 teaspoons coarse ground black pepper. • 3 teaspoons of dill weed. • 2 Tablespoons of smoked paprika.

Combine all your seasoning into your jar and stir before each use for the best flavor and enjoy.

From contributor P. Joines RN, BSN

"Every time you eat or drink, you're either feeding disease or fighting it."

HEATHER MORGAN

MONITORING YOUR FLUID INTAKE

A fluid restriction is put in place to limit the fluid your body retains. When there is excess fluid in your body, your heart has to work harder to maintain blood and oxygen flow, which is necessary for optimal organ function.

The cardiologist will determine the amount of fluid restriction based on the severity of heart failure. It could be as low as 500 mL or as high as 2000 mL per day. Where most people fail in managing their heart failure is adhering to their fluid restriction primarily because it is common to only think about what you drink as fluid intake rather than about what you eat. But all foods that are liquid in form, such as soups and sauces, juicy fruits and vegetables, basically, any food that becomes liquid when melted down, should be counted in your fluid intake.

Some examples would be:

Soups	Yogurt	Cucumbers
Sauces	Salad dressing	Blueberries
Gravies	Gelatin	Cantaloupe
Tomatoes	Celery	Watermelon
Sherbet	Lettuce	Strawberries
Cooked cereal	Pudding	Ice cream

Knowing how many fluid ounces your cup or bowl holds is essential to measuring your fluid intake accurately.

Let's look at some items that you probably use every day.

- The standard coffee cup holds about **eight to ten ounces.**
- Water bottle eight to seventeen ounces.
- Soup/cereal bowl eight to sixteen ounces.
- Standard household cups can hold anywhere from six to thirty-two ounces.

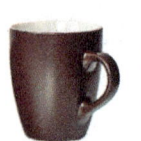

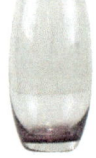

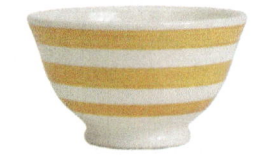

HEART FAILURE AND YOU : A PRACTICAL GUIDE FOR MANAGING YOUR HEART HEALTH

To determine how many fluid ounces your cup or bowl holds:

Set aside a coffee cup, a standard cup, and a bowl from your current dish set.

1. Get a measuring cup, fill it with water, and measure how much fluid each one holds.

2. Grab a sharpie and label the cup and bowl with the number of cups used to fill it and the total number of milliliters (mL) it holds.

3. Another option would be to invest in a measuring cup that includes incremental fluid ounces and milliliters (mL) measurements. You can find these online or at your local discount or craft store.

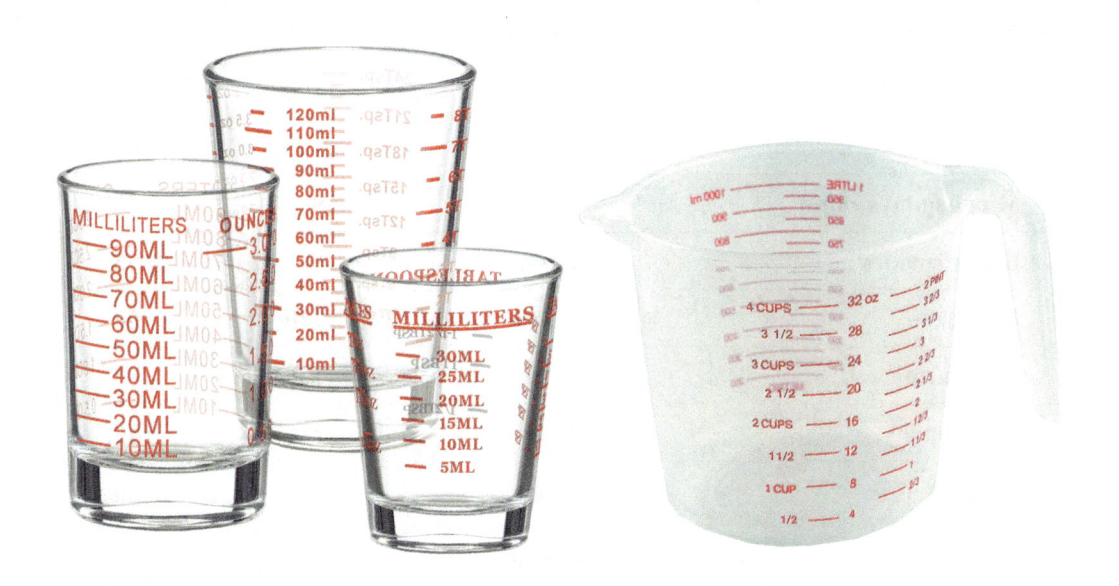

One thing that my family and I found helpful was to create a list of my mom's favorite foods. You can do this by using a marker and paper, and then posting the list on your refrigerator. This way, you will have a quick and easy reference guide to all your favorite foods and beverages with the measurements.

Mom's Fluid and Sodium restriction			
8am to 11pm	1000 mL 800g (2gm)		
What she likes to eat from day to day. Make sure your count what you give her so that she doesn't go over what is allotted for the day.			
Coffee	½ cup	120	0
w/half and half	2 tbl sp	30	15
Bottle of coke	16.9oz	500	65
Bottle of water	16.9oz	500	0
Oatmeal	½ cup	120	0
Mini bag-lays chips	1oz	0	170
Butter cookies	5 cookies	0	95
Ice cream	½ cup	120	53
watermelon	¼ cup	140	0
Jello cup	1 cup	226	40
Jasmine rice	1 cup	0	200
Steamable bag- broccoli cheese	½ cup	70	160
Steamable bag-honey carrots	½ cup	70	85
Steamable bag-sweet corn	2/3 cup	158	20
Turkey sandwich			
Bread	2 slices	0	220
Deli sliced turkey breast	3 slices	0	490
Miracle whip	1 tbl sp	15	95
Mustard	1 tsp	5	60

Another tip would be to divide your daily fluid and sodium restriction into four parts: breakfast, lunch, dinner, and snacks. For instance, if your daily limits are 1000 mL fluid and 800 mg sodium, set a specific amount for each meal. This will help you keep track of your intake and stay within your limits.

Ex.

Breakfast	**240 mL**	**140 mg**
Lunch	**240 mL**	**220 mg**
Dinner	**240 mL**	**220 mg**
Snacks	**280 mL**	**220 mg**

*mL for your fluid intake and mg for your sodium intake.

FLUID CONVERSION TABLE

Fluids	Ounces	mL
2 tablespoons	1 oz	30 mL
1 cup	8 oz	240 mL
1 cup	4 oz	120 mL
1 can of soda	12 oz	360 mL
1 bottle of soda or water	16.9 oz	500 mL
4 cups or 1 quart	32 oz	960 mL
6 cups or 1 ½ quarts	48 oz	1440 mL
8 cups or 2 quarts	64 oz	1920 mL
1 liter	34 oz	1000 mL
Cooked cereal 1/2 cup	4 oz	120 mL
Berries 1 cup	4.6 oz	138 mL
Cucumber slices 1 cup	3.3 oz	100 mL
Shredded lettuce 1 cup	1.5 oz	45 mL
Chicken noodle soup 1 cup	7.5 oz	222 mL
Cottage cheese 1 cup	4 oz	117 mL
Spaghetti sauce 1/2 cup	4 oz	120 mL
Ice cream 1/2 cup	4.0 oz	120 mL
Jell-O 1/2 cup	3.8 oz	113 mL
Pudding 1 cup	3.25 oz	108 mL
Yogurt, 6oz container	4.3 oz	128 mL
Tomato, 3 medium slices	2 oz	57 mL
1 popsicle	1.75 oz	52 mL
Watermelon 1 cup	4.7 oz	140 mL
Cooked broccoli 1 cup	4.7 oz	140 mL
Creamed corn 1 cup	4.7 oz	140 mL

SODIUM CONVERSION TABLE

Sodium	Metric Unit	Mg
Bread	2 slices	220 mg
Deli turkey lunch meat	3 slices	490 mg
Jasmine rice	1 cup	200 mg
Brown rice	1 cup	115 mg
Lays chips (reg)	1 oz bag	170 mg
1 cup of popcorn (popped)	1 cup	65 mg
Spaghetti sauce	1/2 cup	47 mg
Alfredo sauce	1/4 cup	410 mg
Jello	1 cup	40 mg
Pudding	1 cup	120 mg
Vanilla ice cream	1/2 cup	53 mg
Coca Cola	1 bottle (16.9oz)	65 mg
Pepsi	1 bottle (16.9oz)	45 mg
Dr. Pepper	1 bottle (16.9oz)	80 mg
Half and Half	2 tbl spoons	15 mg
Eggs	1 egg	70 mg
American cheese	1 slice	230 mg
Mayonnaise	1 tbl spoon	70 mg
Miracle Whip	1 tbl spoon	95 mg
Ketchup	1 tbl spoon	160 mg
Mustard	1 teaspoon	60 mg
Barbecue Sauce	2 tbl spoons	340 mg
Frozen vegetables (unsauced)	1 cup	10-15 mg
Margarine	1 tbl spoon	90 mg

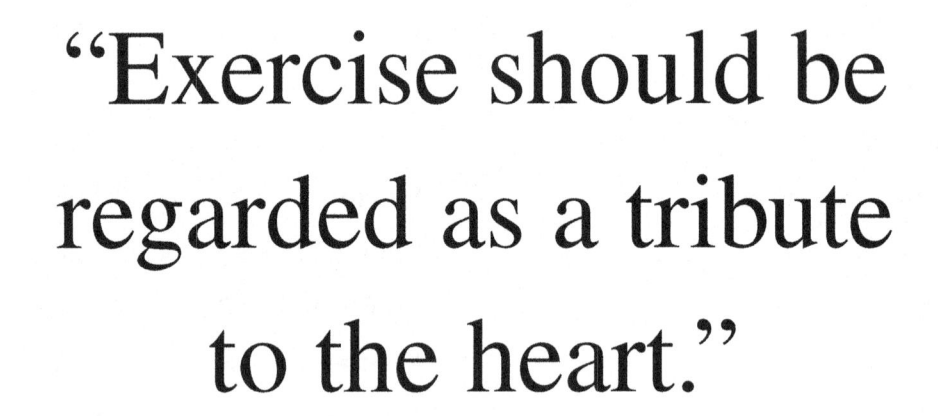

"Exercise should be regarded as a tribute to the heart."

GENE TUNNEY

CHAPTER 3

WORKING OUT FOR YOUR HEART

Exercise is critical after you've received a diagnosis of heart failure. The heart is a muscle, and just like all the other 600 muscles in the body, it requires exercise to keep it healthy and strong. You don't have to go out and run a marathon or spend hours at the gym. You may not even be able to go for a run or a walk. The key is just to get your body moving. Not only will your heart and brain thank you for it, but so will your lungs, digestive system, and mental health. In essence, your whole body will benefit from having a daily exercise routine. So, get active and stay active!

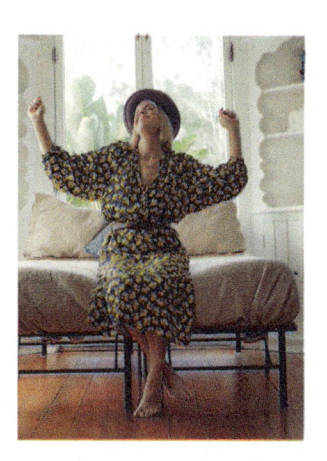

You lose water when you exhale, and your body can lose up to two ounces of water when exercising.

You can do several exercises right in the comfort of your home. For example, put your favorite song on and start moving. Walk around your house for two or three minutes four to five times a day. Dancing, house cleaning; it all counts. The key here is to stay active.

Stretching and yoga are not just for meditation or body alignment. Warming up with basic yoga moves and stretches warms and loosens your muscles and increases blood flow, which can help to decrease muscle injury.

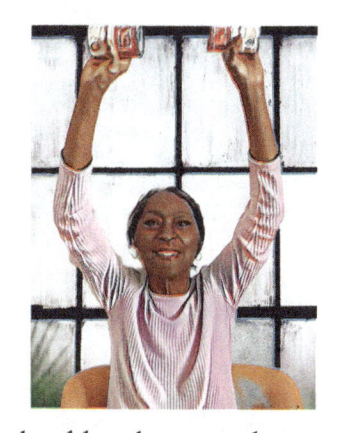

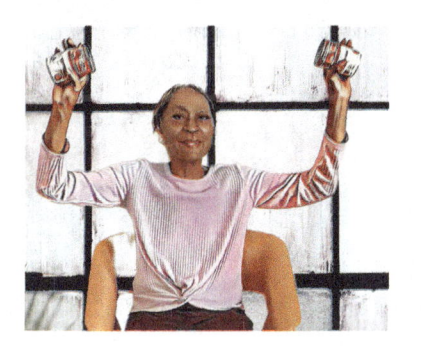

The hokey pokey and head-shoulders-knees-and toes are two must-haves to add to your music playlist. They are an excellent option for a five to ten-minute chair exercise. When done daily, it will help to improve and maintain circulation in your arms and legs. And if you want to add a little weight to your routine, grab two cans of soup from your pantry and use them as your hand weights.

BE SURE TO EXERCISE SAFELY AND LISTEN TO YOUR BODY.

It's normal for your muscles to feel slightly sore for a few days after your first day of exercise, especially if you haven't worked out in a while. However, as you continue to exercise regularly, your muscles will become stronger, and the soreness will eventually go away. If you're still experiencing soreness after a week or if you notice any unusual symptoms, don't hesitate to contact your healthcare team. You know your body better than anyone else.

Know the heart attack warning signs

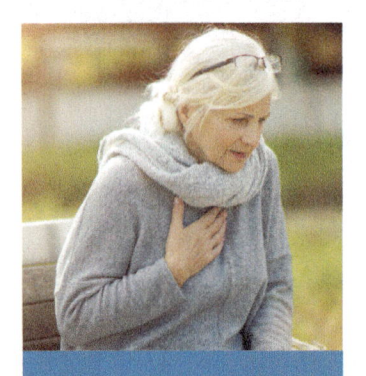

Your chest may hurt or feel squeezed, or it may feel like heartburn or indigestion.

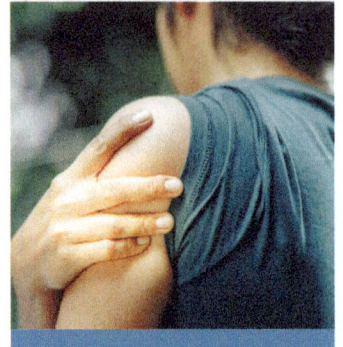

Your arms, back, shoulders, neck, jaw, or upper stomach (above the belly button) may hurt.

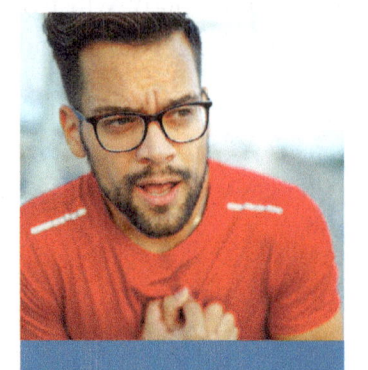

You may feel like you can't breathe.

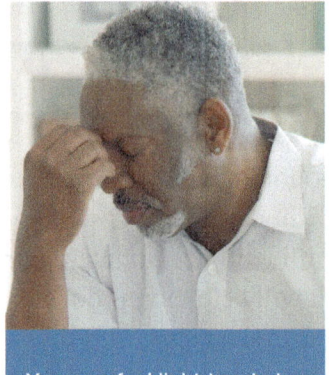

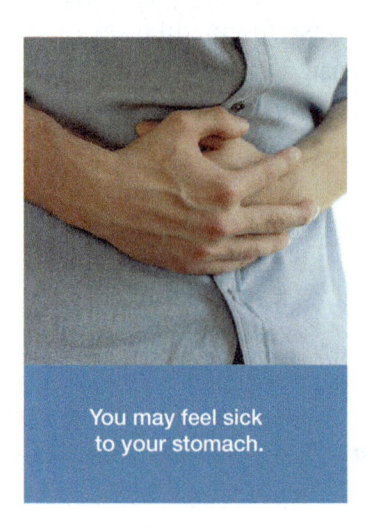

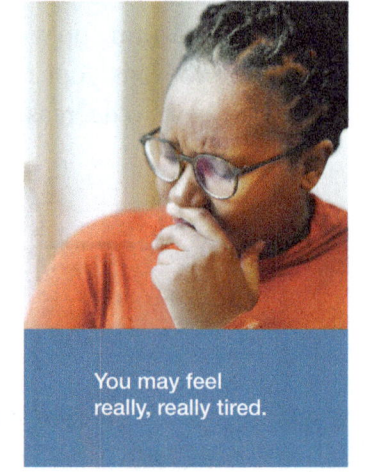

You may feel light-headed or break out in a cold sweat.

You may feel sick to your stomach.

You may feel really, really tired.

(NIH Publication No. 20-HL-5062 2020)

"Take care of your body, it's the only place you have to live."

JIM ROHN

BLOOD PRESSURE AND WEIGHT

Being diagnosed with heart failure also comes with a set of rules and guidelines that require you to be as organized and detailed as possible. You'll need to follow a specific schedule to track and log your blood pressure, weight, fluid intake, sodium intake, and, for some of you, how much urine you put out.

You should check your blood pressure at least twice daily, morning and evening, and your weight in the mornings. However, this may vary based on the instructions given to you by your provider.

Monitoring Your Blood Pressure

Some insurance carriers will cover the cost of a blood pressure monitor when prescribed by your doctor. If you have to or plan to purchase a blood pressure monitor, here are a few things you should know;

- Avoid the wrist monitor, as the readings from these monitors tend not to be as accurate as an arm monitor.
- Be sure to choose a monitor that has been validated. You can get help from the pharmacist or check online at validatebp.org before purchasing.
- Most importantly, ensure your monitor has the right cuff size for your arm.

You always want to ensure you get accurate blood pressure readings from your monitor. So, here are a few things that can cause false blood pressure readings that you should know about.

1. **Wrong size blood pressure cuff.** A blood pressure cuff that is too big or too small can cause your blood pressure to read higher or lower than it is.
2. **Improper positioning.** Sitting with your legs crossed at the knee will increase your blood pressure reading.
3. **Incorrect placement of the cuff.** The cuff should be placed on the upper arm, above the elbow, with the tubing over the center of the arm; you should be sitting upright with the arm relaxed at the side.

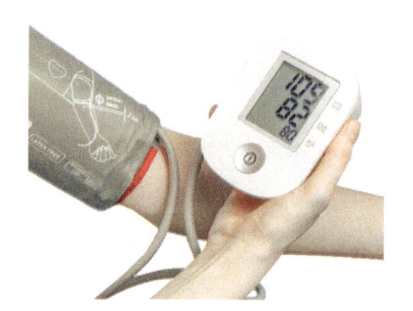

TRACKING YOUR WEIGHT

To measure your weight accurately, you can buy a digital or analog scale online or from a local store. You can find one for around $10-$15. After getting the scale, ensure that it is placed on a flat and even surface, and calibrate it by zeroing it out before using it.

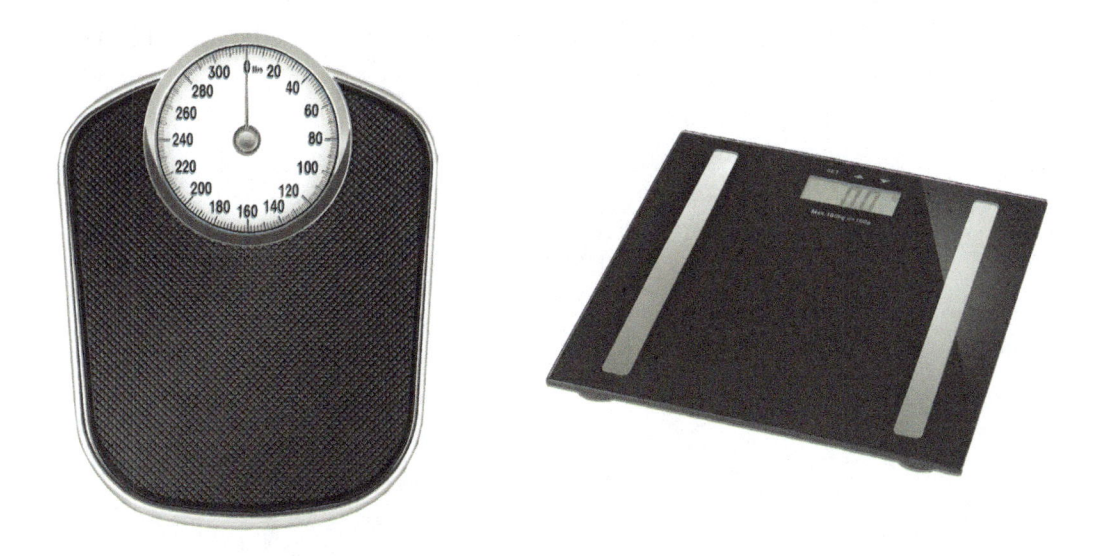

To get the most precise reading, weigh yourself in the morning when you wake up. This is the best time as you don't have to account for the food you've eaten or hormone changes throughout the day that can affect your weight.

It is crucial to weigh yourself in the same way and at the same time every day. For instance, if you wear pajamas and slippers the first time you weigh yourself, then you should wear the same outfit every time to prevent your weight from being altered by what you're wearing. Note that to get the most accurate reading, it is best to weigh yourself without clothes.

Notify your provider's office if you have an increase in your weight by two pounds in twenty-four hours or five pounds in a week. The weight gain could signify that you are retaining fluid. And this calls for a visit to the doctor. You don't want your heart to work any harder than it has to, and excess fluid in the body increases the heart's workload. So, getting the extra weight gain decreased and resolved as soon as possible is imperative to prevent any health complications. The treatment option could be as simple as adjusting your medication dosage, adding another medication like a diuretic, or scheduling another consult with the dietician.

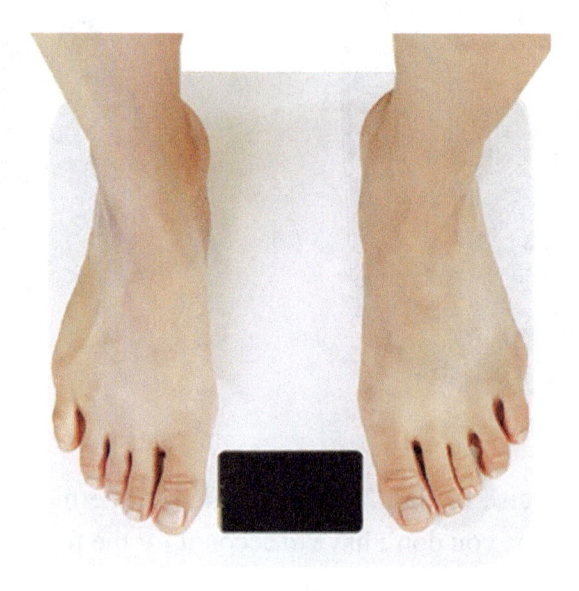

RED FLAGS

Below is a list of common signs and symptoms that you are carrying more fluid in your body than your heart can manage, and it's time to give your doctor's office a call.

- Have you gained five pounds or more over a period of two or three days?
- Do you feel bloated?
- Look at the veins in your neck; do they look bigger?
- Do you get short of breath after walking from room to room?
- Are you more tired (fatigue) than usual?
- Are you more comfortable sleeping while sitting up than lying down?
- Are you having chest pain or feeling pressure like something is sitting on your chest?
- Do you feel like your heart is racing or skipping a beat?
- Do you hear your heart beating in your ear?
- Do you feel dizzy, confused, or have a headache that just won't go away?
- Do your legs look swollen (bigger) or feel heavier than usual?
- When you press your finger to your skin, does your finger leave what we call a pit or indentation?
- Does your skin look tight or shiny?
- Do you feel like you are going to the bathroom less than usual?
- These are all individual signs you need to seek medical attention immediately.

General tip: When calling your doctor's office or going to the emergency room, remember to be specific and describe what and how you are feeling. Tell them what you felt, where you felt it, how long it lasted, if it moved from one area of your body to another, what you were doing before it started, and if you tried anything to relieve the symptoms before notifying them.

CONCLUSION

Whoever coined the phrase "there are no dumb questions" was right. Asking questions is key to gaining knowledge and understanding.

*When you have heart disease,
knowledge is the power that can save your life!*

Silence has no place in the doctor's office unless a stethoscope is involved. So, don't be afraid, feel intimidated, or, more importantly, be in too much of a hurry to get out of the exam room to strike up a conversation with the doctor and ask questions.

Your provider is concerned with how you're feeling, thinking, and how you're taking care of yourself. So, all of the thoughts that keep you up at night, the ones you ponder over while having your morning cup of coffee, even the ones that you didn't think about but you read on the cover of a magazine in the grocery store, we want to hear about them. These conversations help ensure you get quality healthcare mentally, physically, and emotionally.

It's better to ask a hundred questions during your visit than to leave without understanding how to manage your new medications, diagnosis, or changes in your condition. Your questions are essential not only for your benefit but also for your healthcare team.

To make the most out of each appointment, it's a good idea to create a list of questions beforehand. Take note of any feedback about your medication routine and be prepared to discuss what's working and what's not working for you. You should also add a list of things you want to try; you might introduce your healthcare team to something new.

And if, for any reason, you don't feel comfortable with your provider, contact your insurance company and find one that you do feel comfortable with. Managing your health is a team effort, and you should feel comfortable with everyone on your team. At the end of the day, this is your life that you are advocating for. **So, speak up!**

"Knowledge is power, and it can help you overcome any fear of the unexpected. When you learn, you gain more awareness through the process, and you know what pitfalls to look for as you get ready to transition to the next level."

JAY SHETTY

Thank you for reading my book!

In the pages that follow you will find a personal information page. A medical information and medication page. There is also a four-week log to monitor and track your daily blood pressure, weight, fluid, and sodium intake.

On the log sheet, you will find an area to note the month and year, date, and standard time frames for blood pressure checks, boxes to enter your fluid and sodium intake, and a box for your weight and the time you weighed. There is also an additional box to note your urine output for the day should you be required to measure it as well.

Ex.

Date	Blood pressure		Fluids (mL)	Sodium (mg)	Weight	Time	Time Urine Output for the day
4/18	7am -9am	132/90	975	485	115	815am	1200
	12am -2pm	124/87					
	7pm -9pm	123/88					

PERSONAL INFORMATION

Name

Address

City **State** **Zip**

Phone **Cell**

E-mail

In Case of Emergency

1st Notify **Relationship**

Phone **Cell**

In Case of Emergency

2nd Notify **Relationship**

Phone **Cell**

MEDICAL INFORMATION

Allergies

Blood Type

Doctor 1
Name

Phone

Specialty

Doctor 2
Name

Phone

Specialty

Doctor 3
Name

Phone

Specialty

Doctor 4
Name

Phone

Specialty

MEDICATIONS

Name	Dosage	Frequency	Notes:
Ex: Coumadin	3mg	1x a day	1 tab on Sun/Th and 1/2 tab the other days

1st WEEK

Date	Blood pressure	Fluids (mL)	Sodium (mg)	Weight	Time	Time Urine Output for the day
	7am -9am / 12am -2pm / 7pm -9pm					
	7am -9am / 12am -2pm / 7pm -9pm					
	7am -9am / 12am -2pm / 7pm -9pm					
	7am -9am / 12am -2pm / 7pm -9pm					
	7am -9am / 12am -2pm / 7pm -9pm					
	7am -9am / 12am -2pm / 7pm -9pm					
	7am -9am / 12am -2pm / 7pm -9pm					

2nd WEEK

Date	Blood pressure		Fluids (mL)	Sodium (mg)	Weight	Time	Time Urine Output for the day
	7am -9am 12am -2pm 7pm -9pm						
	7am -9am 12am -2pm 7pm -9pm						
	7am -9am 12am -2pm 7pm -9pm						
	7am -9am 12am -2pm 7pm -9pm						
	7am -9am 12am -2pm 7pm -9pm						
	7am -9am 12am -2pm 7pm -9pm						
	7am -9am 12am -2pm 7pm -9pm						

3rd WEEK

Date	Blood pressure	Fluids (mL)	Sodium (mg)	Weight	Time	Time Urine Output for the day
	7am -9am 12am -2pm 7pm -9pm					
	7am -9am 12am -2pm 7pm -9pm					
	7am -9am 12am -2pm 7pm -9pm					
	7am -9am 12am -2pm 7pm -9pm					
	7am -9am 12am -2pm 7pm -9pm					
	7am -9am 12am -2pm 7pm -9pm					
	7am -9am 12am -2pm 7pm -9pm					

4th WEEK

Date	Blood pressure	Fluids (mL)	Sodium (mg)	Weight	Time	Time Urine Output for the day
	7am -9am 12am -2pm 7pm -9pm					
	7am -9am 12am -2pm 7pm -9pm					
	7am -9am 12am -2pm 7pm -9pm					
	7am -9am 12am -2pm 7pm -9pm					
	7am -9am 12am -2pm 7pm -9pm					
	7am -9am 12am -2pm 7pm -9pm					
	7am -9am 12am -2pm 7pm -9pm					

Date	Blood pressure	Fluids (mL)	Sodium (mg)	Weight	Time	Time Urine Output for the day
	7am -9am 12am -2pm 7pm -9pm					
	7am -9am 12am -2pm 7pm -9pm					
	7am -9am 12am -2pm 7pm -9pm					
	7am -9am 12am -2pm 7pm -9pm					
	7am -9am 12am -2pm 7pm -9pm					
	7am -9am 12am -2pm 7pm -9pm					
	7am -9am 12am -2pm 7pm -9pm					

"Life isn't a matter of milestones, but of moments."

ROSE KENNEDY

NOTES

NOTES

NOTES

NOTES

NOTES

NOTES

NOTES

NOTES

NOTES

NOTES

NOTES

NOTES

NOTES

NOTES

REFERENCES

n.d. " Get Involved Ways to Give." American Heart Association. Accessed February 11, 2023.
https://www.heart.org/en/get-involved/ways-to-give?s_src=23I711AEMG&s_subsrc=fy23_mar_sem_google_text&utm_medium=paid&utm_campaign=dr+fy23+march-match&utm_source=sem+google&utm_content=prospecting-remarketing+sem+evergreensem&utm_term=text&gclid=Cj0KCQiAj.

Antipolis, Sophia. 2020. "Poor diet is top contributor to heart disease deaths globally." European Society of Cardiology. October 16. Accessed March 7, 2023.
https://www.escardio.org/The-ESC/Press-Office/Press-releases/poor-diet-is-top-contributor-to-heart-disease-deaths-globally.

2020. "FAST Poster 2020." American Stroke Association. Accessed March 3, 2023.
https://www.stroke.org/en/help-and-support/resource-library/fast-materials/fast-poster-2020.

2023. "Heart Failure." Centers for Disease Control and Prevention. January 5. Accessed January 13, 2023.
https://www.cdc.gov/heartdisease/heart_failure.htm.

Jayan, Dr. Nithin. 2019. " Congestive Heart Failure ." Medindia. "Congestive Heart Failure Current Management ". December 12. Accessed January 29, 2023.
https://www.medindia.net/patients/patientinfo/congestive-heart-failure.htm.

Jillian Kubala, MS, RD. 2021. "6 Fantastic Health Benefits of Greek Yogurt." Healthline. 10 27. Accessed 3 5, 2023.
https://www.healthline.com/health/food-nutrition/greek-yogurt-benefits#what-it-is.

Karthikeyan Ananth, M.D. 2019. "How Laughter Benefits Your Heart Health." Henry Ford Health. March 5. Accessed January 29, 2023.
https://www.henryford.com/blog/2019/03/how-laughter-benefits-heart-health#:~:text=When%20you%20laugh%2C%20your%20heart,of%20a%20heart%20disease%20diagnosis.

NIH Publication No. 20-HL-5062. 2020. "Learn What a Heart Attack Feels Like." National Heart, Lung, and Blood Institute. October. Accessed March 3, 2023.
https://www.nhlbi.nih.gov/resources/learn-what-heart-attack-feels.

2020. "Recipes and Nutrition." American Diabetes Association. February. Accessed March 12, 2023.
https://www.diabetesfoodhub.org/articles/what-is-the-diabetes-plate-method.html#:~:text=The%20Diabetes%20Plate%20Method%20is,you%20need%20is%20a%20plate!

Watson, Stephanie, and RD, LD Christine Mikstas. n.d. "Do Air Fryers Have Health Benefits?" WebM.
https://www.webmd.com/food-recipes/air-fryers#:~:text=By%20most%20measures%2C%20air%20frying,harmful%20effects%20of%20oil%20frying.

n.d. "When Should I Call 911?" Parkwest Medical Center Covenant Health. Accessed March 3, 2023.
https://www.treatedwell.com/er/when-should-i-call-911/.

Images & illustrations credits:

- Pixabay.com
- Freepik.com
- IStock: Analog scale- Daneger
- IStock: Digital scale- Marcelo Trad
- IStock: Chicken meal prep dish- YelenaYemchuk